How To Whiten Your Teeth

322 Great Teeth Whitening Tips For Beautiful White Teeth Smiles

ADAM COLTON

Published by BizMove
www.bizmove.com

322 Great Teeth Whitening Tips For Beautiful white teeth Smiles

You will not find a better collection of teeth whitening tips elsewhere, so stop searching and read what we have to give you. Everything in this book is free for you to use and provided by experts in the subject that want to make sure everybody has a beautiful smile.

1. Try not to drink water that contains fluoride or using any toothpaste that contains it. Contrary to the popular belief that it is good for your teeth it has been shown to have a staining effect! Other countries have all together banned the use of it in their water because of dangers.

2. When thinking about whitening your teeth, it is important to keep in mind the color of your natural teeth. Whitening will give you the best results if you have yellow teeth. If your teeth are brownish you will receive medium results. Whitening is least affective on teeth that are gray in color.

3. When trying to whiten your teeth, use toothpaste specifically made for teeth whitening. These toothpastes use peroxides that act as a bleaching agent for your teeth. Be sure to look at the

amount of peroxide in the toothpaste, typically the concentration is between ten and twenty percent. Choose a product in the middle, and if your teeth tolerate the toothpaste (and you want more effective whitening), move up to a toothpaste with 20% peroxide.

4. Teeth whitening may seem like a very difficult task, but when you follow a few basic tips it can be very simple. One of the most important things to do when it comes to improving your tooth color is to avoid things that will make it worse, such as the things found in this article.

5. When you whiten your teeth, the crowns will not whiten as well as your teeth do. If you have visible crowns, your teeth can present themselves as unevenly colored. Consult with your dental professional for ways to minimize this problem.

6. Along with being high in sugar and/or high fructose corn syrup, wine and soda can stain your teeth. That makes these beverages a double hazard for your teeth. Avoid these beverages or rinse your mouth out with water after drinking soda or wine, better yet, brush your teeth if possible.

7. Baking soda is great for whitening teeth, plus, it is inexpensive and easy to get. Purchase tooth paste with baking soda in it for extra whitening every day. You can also make your own whitening paste by mixing baking soda with a pinch of salt. Rub this paste on your teeth, let it sit for a few minutes and then brush as usual.

8. If you are trying to get whiter teeth, you should have regular dental cleaning appointments. Your teeth will be noticeably whiter as a result of cleaning by your dental hygienist. You should go to your dentist for cleanings at least two times a year.

9. For the whitest and cleanest teeth possible, invest in an effective electric tooth brush. The more expensive models of electric toothbrushes can help brush your teeth more effectively than humanly possible with a manual toothbrush. Make sure you invest in a rechargeable electric toothbrush with replaceable heads for the best value.

10. Some fruits can naturally whiten your teeth. Strawberries are great for whitening. You can rub them on your teeth or mash them up into a paste, brush them on, and leave them for about five minutes. Rinse your teeth well. Orange peel

is also good for whitening. You can rub it directly on the teeth. Another natural fruit tooth whitener is lemon juice and salt mixed together.

11. Use toothpaste meant for teeth whitening. You can also buy special floss that will whiten your teeth as you use it. Any tooth related product that contains baking soda will be a valuable tool in your teeth whitening endeavors, as it is a good stain remover.

12. Drink fewer soft drinks. These drinks have dyes in them that can cause your teeth to become discolored. Other soda ingredients can really harm the enamel on the teeth. When the enamel is damaged, stains sink in deeper and get harder to deal with. Too many of these drinks will make your teeth harder to whiten if you drink them regularly.

13. Flossing your teeth is very important. Flossing regularly helps rid the plaque buildup on your teeth which is one of the causes of discoloration. Keep a single-use toothbrush and floss in your wallet or purse for cleaning while you're away from home. You should also floss at the end of the day so the bacterias do not get a chance to damage your teeth during the night.

14. Make a paste containing baking soda and hydrogen peroxide and use it to brush teeth. Using gently strokes, brush teeth with this combination to create whiter teeth, while avoiding chemicals that can have a negative effect. Make sure that you do not swallow any of the mixture. If you were to drink this by accident, you should immediately drink a few cups of water.

15. Talk with your dentist before beginning any teeth whitening program. If you currently have any sort of dental disease or issue, your dentist may recommend a specific method of teeth whitening. Most natural remedies do not have side effects, but if you are prone to gum problems or teeth sensitivity, some remedies may not be appropriate.

16. When you drink something, use a straw. A lot of beverages will discolor your teeth, so try to drink them using a straw. If you try to minimize your teeth's contact with these drinks, you can have a smile that is whiter.

17. While some advocates of home remedies to whiten teeth recommend making toothpaste from mashed strawberries and baking soda, this can actually be detrimental to your teeth.

Strawberries contain malic acid, which can whiten your teeth. However, the flip side is that it can also erode the enamel. Strawberries also contain natural sugars that can harm the teeth. A much safer alternative is to eat an apple. If you don't have a toothbrush on hand, an apple can help to remove surface stains and break down any remaining food particles in the mouth. Apples also contain a small amount of malic acid, but you would have to eat an unrealistic amount of them for it to do any damage.

18. If you are trying to whiten your teeth try to increase the frequency with which you brush your teeth. For exampleif you are currently brushing once or twice daily try to increase it to two or there times daily focusing on times especially after meals and snacks. This will help whiten your smile.

19. You are going to damage your teeth in a way that cannot be repaired if you over treat your teeth with teeth whitening gels or pastes. Only use them as they are directed on the label of the brand that you are using. You will avoid doing damage to your teeth when trying to get them white.

20. Do not start a home teeth whitening treatment without going to the dentist to have an exam done. You do not want to use any of these treatments if you have untreated cavities in your mouth. The same goes for gum disease. These things should be treated prior to any treatment.

21. Your dentist may be willing to advise you about what home whitening kits will work the best without causing damage to your teeth or your gums. There are some systems that work on some people but not others, ask your dentist.

22. When you want whiter teeth in a hurry, grab an apple to eat for a temporary solution. The consistency of the apple has the ability to scrape off food, which gives your teeth a cleaner appearance in just a few bites.

23. Always follow the directions exactly as they are printed when using teeth whiteners. If you put these things on your teeth and leave them on longer than directed, you might see some damage. Stay away from drinks with acidic ingredients, such as sports drinks or sodas, after using a whitening product. This is an extra protective measure to ensure that no harmful reactions occur.

24. When you have reached the level of whitening that you want on your teeth, be sure to stop and go into maintenance mode! Because of the affordability of many teeth whitening products, it's very tempting just to keep going. In this instance, more is not better! You can seriously damage your teeth with ongoing usage. At this point, do the whitening sessions only once or twice every year.

25. To maintain the results of your whitening, stay away from cigarettes and processed foods. Teeth friendly foods like apples, celery, and carrots will keep your teeth healthy and bright. Chewing on a sugar free gum can also be very helpful, as it stimulates the production of saliva, which can lead to a cleaner mouth.

26. If you are in need of a whiter, brighter smile, then you try rubbing wood ash on your teeth! Amazingly, wood ash contains content that will help to bleach your teeth. Additionally, wood ash is coarse to it helps to scrap off excess plaque on the surface of your teeth.

27. Before starting a teeth whitening treatment, be aware that whiteners work only on natural teeth. Dental devices such as veneers, crowns or implants will stay their current shade. If you

whiten your teeth even though you have some dental work may not be a good idea, because the dental work will not whiten.

28. One of the primary causes of having discolored teeth and smile in general is bad habits with beverages. Coffee is one of the leading causes of having teeth that are discolored. If you are determined to continue drinking coffee then you will want to brush your teeth immediately after each cup.

29. To help whiten your teeth, chew gum often after meals. Your teeth are naturally white and certain gums enable the mouth to do its own biochemistry and whitening and preservation of enamel after a meal. To get the most out of your teeth whitening efforts, let the body do all it can before you hit the toothpaste.

30. Eat crunchy vegetables like apples and celery to help remove surface stains on your teeth. Think of them as like a loofah for your smile. They exfoliate the teeth before the stains can get deeply attached to the surface of your teeth. Fibrous foods like spinach, lettuce and broccoli will also work.

31. Learn to brush properly to get a whiter smile. You should be holding your toothbrush at a 45-degree angle against your gums and then using a circular motion to brush your teeth with instead of the back and forward motion you were taught. To make sure you don't scrub too hard, hold the brush like you would a pencil.

32. Prevention of staining is one way to keep your teeth whiter. Some of the things you drink can cause discoloration of your teeth. Coffee, tea, wine and soda are all notorious for causing stains on teeth. If you will sip them or drink them through a straw this will help them to not make as much contact with your teeth. Also, when you are done with your drink, rinse your mouth with water.

33. If you are getting metal braces you should use a tooth whitener prior to getting them. Doing this will make your teeth look much whiter once the braces are removed. No question that your new smile will make you happier.

34. Before you commit to a certain over-the-counter teeth whitener, you may want to check online reviews or ask your friends for their experience with it. Many times, people pay ridiculous amounts for a product that promises to whiten

their teeth, when in reality, it does absolutely nothing to help or makes teeth color worse.

35. To make your teeth whitening results last as long as possible, cut back on your consumption of dark drinks like colas and coffee. Since most teeth whitening treatments strip away a layer of your tooth enamel, your teeth are more susceptible than ever to stains, making it more important than ever that you refrain from indulging in common staining culprits like soda, coffee and cigarettes.

36. Try not to drink water that contains fluoride or using any toothpaste that contains it. Contrary to the popular belief that it is good for your teeth it has been shown to have a staining effect! Other countries have all together banned the use of it in their water because of dangers.

37. To have a white smile, make sure you avoid drinking water or using toothpastes that contain fluoride. It has been reported that fluoride may aid in discoloring and permanently staining your teeth. Many countries have actually banned fluoride from their drinking water due to this very reason. To stay on the safe side, avoid fluoride at all costs for a healthy and white smile.

38. Approximately half of all patients who try some sort of whitening treatment, especially those at home, will experience some level of tooth sensitivity as a result. If this happens to you, try lowering the concentration of the product that you are using, and see if that corrects the problem.

39. Do not use teeth bleaching or whitening kits if you are pregnant. Swallowing even a trace amount of the chemicals and ingredients in these kits is enough to potentially cause harm to the fetus. Instead make sure that you wait until after your baby is born to try a teeth whitening program.

40. When you have reached the level of whitening that you want on your teeth, be sure to stop and go into maintenance mode! Because of the affordability of many teeth whitening products, it's very tempting just to keep going. In this instance, more is not better! You can seriously damage your teeth with ongoing usage. At this point, do the whitening sessions only once or twice every year.

41. If you're pregnant, avoid any teeth whitening method that involves bleaching. The bleach could potentially have harmful effects on your

baby. But, there are other issues as well. Teeth are more sensitive during pregnancy, and a harsh treatment that your teeth could normally handle may be incredibly painful. Try a whitening toothpaste or natural whitening methods until after you have your baby.

42. Two great fruits to help you naturally whiten your teeth are pears and apples. When eaten, both of these fruits create a large amount of saliva. The additional saliva helps clean those stained teeth. So next time you are looking for a healthy snack, choose one that will also whiten your teeth!

43. Another great way to keep your teeth looking good is to start drinking all of your fluids through a straw. This minimizes contact with your teeth, which helps to minimize the discoloration of your teeth caused by drinking colored fluids. This is an easy way to avoid discoloration.

44. You should not begin a teeth whitening regiment until you are around the age of 16 to 18. Until this time a child's gums are incredibly sensitive. Therefore, the caustic and abrasive products that are used to clean teeth can cause a child's mouth to enter a world of pain.

45. If you are using a peroxide treatment to keep up your beautiful smile, then you need to make sure that you do not over do it. These treatments should be applied once every 6 to 8 months. Any more than this can cause damage to your gums and your teeth.

46. Make sure to contact your dentist before starting to use an over the counter tooth whitening treatment. No one wants to wait for whiter teeth, but discoloration could be a sign of a more serious issue. Take the time to let your doctor rule out any issues and then whiten away.

47. As the famous saying goes, "An apple a day keeps the doctor away". This includes dentists. Apples are crisp and smooth when you bite into them and biting an apple actually cleans your teeth. Apples also contain properties that can kill most of the bacteria that sits on your teeth.

48. To help prevent your teeth from getting stained, try to stay away from foods and drinks that are known to stain your teeth. Avoid foods like blueberries and soy sauce. In moderation, these foods are okay, but try not to over do it. Drinks like tea and coffee will also cause stains on your teeth.

49. You should not smoke cigarettes. Smoking can cause unsightly stains on your pearly whites and is potentially disastrous to your health. People who smoke frequently have yellowed teeth. It can be rather difficult to keep a bright white smile if you smoke. If quitting smoking is not an option, cut back as much as possible for the sake of your health and to have a white, bright smile.

50. A great way to naturally whiten your teeth without resorting to harsh chemicals is to use a lemon juice and salt mixture. Using this mixture as a mouthwash is a cheap and effective way that way to remove surface stains from your teeth. Be sure to rinse with water afterward.

51. If you have a large number of enhancements on your teeth, such as crowns, veneers, implants, and fillings, tooth whitening procedures are probably not a good idea. This is because the chemicals used to whiten your teeth will only work on the natural tooth surface, and you'll be left with a patchwork effect.

52. Rather than focusing on removing stains from your teeth with whitening pastes, creams and gels, why not avoid staining them in the first place? Coffee and tea are notorious for staining

teeth and should be avoided if at all possible. If you do drink them, try rinsing your mouth out with clean water when you are done to minimize staining.

53. Once you go through the teeth whitening treatment, you are going to want to avoid drinking things or eating foods that are known to stain teeth. Newly whitened teeth are prone to absorbing the staining agents that are in these things and you may find yourself worse off than before you treated your teeth.

54. In order to get white teeth a good habit that you can do is to choose to eat food that naturally whitens teeth. Examples of these are raw fruits and vegetables that scrub your teeth while you eat them. These foods include carrots, strawberries, apples, celery, pineapples, oranges and pears.

55. To keep your teeth white, be sure to use a straw when you are drinking beverages with high levels of acidity. The acidity in beverages, like sodas or sports drinks, can affect the color of your teeth, but the straw acts as a barrier. This will not change the color of your teeth overnight and if your teeth are already stained it will not take off

the stain. It will help to prevent more discoloration.

56. For inexpensive teeth whitening at home, brush your teeth thoroughly and then swish a mouthful of hydrogen peroxide inside your mouth for as long as possible before spitting it out into the sink. Hydrogen peroxide is an active ingredient in most commercial teeth whitening products and provides an oxygenating action that helps lift stains from teeth.

57. Floss your teeth. You should floss thoroughly at least twice a day. Flossing removes food and helps to fight the build-up of plaque. Most people do not bother to floss at all. Neglecting to do so can damage your teeth. To keep them looking their best, remember to floss.

58. When using over the counter teeth whitening products, make sure that you follow the instructions exactly. Some people may try to leave strips or gels on their teeth longer than directed in an effort to enhance or quicken results. This can cause irritation to your gums and result in inflammation. Stick to the directions and exercise patience.

59. Try using some whitening strips to brighten your smile. They actually do work well to lighten your teeth a couple shades. For the best results, it is recommended that you use them at least six hours after brushing. Make sure to dry your teeth with a tissue before you apply the strips.

60. Removing plaque is essential to whitening your teeth and the best method for ridding yourself of plaque is to use an electric toothbrush. Plaque creates a good surface for stains to build on. Electric toothbrushes are recommended by most dentists due to their ability to break up plaque and remove the stains that are associated with it.

61. To help whiten your teeth, chew gum often after meals. Your teeth are naturally white and certain gums enable the mouth to do its own biochemistry and whitening and preservation of enamel after a meal. To get the most out of your teeth whitening efforts, let the body do all it can before you hit the toothpaste.

62. Change your diet for whiter teeth. Avoid processed foods and foods high in sugar. Replace them with lots of raw fruits and vegetables that help clean your teeth while you eat them and promote healthy salivation during

chewing. Not only will this help whiten you teeth, it will also keep them strong and healthy.

63. One important teeth whitening tip is to make sure that you both brush and floss your teeth on a regular basis. This is important for your overall oral health as well as making sure that you are removing anything that will stain or discolor your teeth such as plaque or coffee.

64. Though it is commonly used for this exact purpose, it may not be safe to actually use hydrogen peroxide for the purpose of teeth whitening. Not only is this unsafe, hydrogen peroxide can actually promote discoloration of your teeth. Refrain from using hydrogen peroxide when trying to whiten your teeth.

65. If you want to whiten your teeth, use whitening strips. Whitening strips are very popular and are a simple and quick way to whiten your teeth. Simply stick the strips to your teeth. Let them stay there for several minutes, and then take them off. Repeat this for several days until you get the whitening you desire.

66. One important teeth whitening tip is to make sure that you always drink plenty of water. This will act as a natural way to remove extra food

and harmful materials from your teeth, keeping them whiter. Be sure to rinse with water after eating as often as possible.

67. One important teeth whitening tip is that before you do anything other than natural methods, consult with a professional first. This will ensure that you are not making some sort of mistake that you may regret later in life. You could possibly cause damage to your teeth or waste a lot of money.

68. Keep your mouth healthy and brush and floss at least two times every day. Floss after every meal that you eat if you can. You can buy small disposable hand held flossers that make it easy and discreet. After every time you floss make sure that you rinse out your mouth.

69. Listerine teeth whitening mouthwash rinse is a great product to help you whiten your teeth. Within the first couple of weeks of usage you can easily see the difference in your teeth. Make sure to use twice a day- once in the morning and once at night. Listerine is strong in killing bad breath and whitens your teeth at the same time.

70. Determine why your teeth are discolored before starting any whitening treatment. A trip to your

dentist should answer this question. Knowing the cause of your discolored teeth will give you the best treatment options for your specific problems and therefore you will also get the best results too.

71. Strips for teeth whitening are available at almost every drugstore and are quite affordable. Simply leave the strip on your teeth for the amount of time suggested by the manufacturer. Whitening strips are diminishing in popularity, due to other methods that are much more effective.

72. For many years people have sworn that baking soda works quite well for teeth whitening. There are now many types of toothpaste that have baking soda right in them so you do not have to mess with making up the paste yourself. The paste is made up with a bit of salt and baking soda and then brushed onto your teeth.

73. Use oranges to whiten your teeth. This has been proven to whiten teeth. You can use the peel of an orange to do this. Using the back of the orange peel, put it in your mouth and rub it on the surface of your teeth. Keep it there for about 5 minutes.

74. Be careful and use teeth whitening products exactly as directed. Leaving these products on your teeth longer than the recommended time can have serious ramifications like gum inflammation and increased sensitivity. Avoid drinking anything with a high level of acidity after cleaning your teeth, for instance sodas or energy drinks.

75. If you are in dire need of whiter teeth you can try going to your dentist and getting an in office bleaching. While this may be a little more expensive, this technique is proven to whiten your teeth right away. Get the smile you have always wanted with in office bleaching.

76. It is so important that whenever you get your teeth whitened, after every meal you must brush your teeth. Food can encourage the growth of bacteria in your mouth and on your teeth. Following most whitening treatments, your teeth are especially vulnerable to this bacteria, so you have to be scrupulous about brushing.

77. You should understand that your crowns will never whiten like the rest of your teeth. If you use a whitening technique on your teeth but your crowns which are not whitened show, people will see some of your teeth as white and some

discolored, giving an odd effect. If this is occurring, then having a discussion with your dentist on the best teeth whitening options would be wise, so that the colors remain close to each other.

78. Several dental companies are currently selling different types of strips to place in the mouth and aid in whitening. These are actually one of the best ways to improve your smile outside of a medical procedure. Although they may be a bit expensive they are quite effective and can help a great deal.

79. There are many different companies that offer teeth whitening kits. There are gels, strips and many other types of products. Some of these are definitely worth giving a try if you are having problems with yellowing teeth. Make sure to read the reviews on the various products that are out there, otherwise you could be wasting your money.

80. If you do want to make your teeth look whiter by using lip makeup, opt for brighter reds and oranges for your color choices. Colors like light red and coral can really make your teeth appear whiter, while using colors that are very light can make any yellow in your teeth stand out.

81. Enamel is the protective mineral layer that helps prevent root infections as well as other things that can harm the teeth. Some treatments available in the marketplace are overly acidic and toxic, which can work against you in your efforts to have bright and healthy teeth.

82. One important teeth whitening tip is to make sure that you pay attention to how your teeth react to whitening products. Often times it can make sensitive teeth more sensitive and can cause normal teeth to become more sensitive. This can be very uncomfortable when eating extremely hot or cold food and drinks.

83. If you want whiter teeth, drink lots of water. Water rinses your mouth of harmful bacteria. It also helps to remove stubborn foods that can cause staining. Try to rinse your mouth at least two or three times a day, and drink at least eight glasses of water.

84. There is a lack of evidence suggesting that they are more helpful than regular toothpastes. Talk to your dentist and ask for recommendations of products that give the best results.

85. Rinse your mouth out with 3% hydrogen peroxide solution every evening after you brush your teeth. 3% hydrogen peroxide solution is a mild bleaching agent so it can help to keep your teeth white, it is also very cheap; you should be able to pick up a bottle in your local pharmacy for less than $2.

86. Surprisingly, baking soda is almost as effective as most long term teeth whiteners and is much cheaper. Mix about two table spoons of soda to one table spoon of water to form a paste, then, brush your teeth with this paste. If you do not like the taste, substitute a mouthwash for the water.

87. When you want whiter teeth, do not be fooled by the different kinds of toothpastes available. Toothpaste that claims to whiten your teeth is frequently more expensive than normal toothpaste. When trying to remove stains from your teeth, regular toothpaste works just as well and is often cheaper than whitening toothpaste.

88. If you have oral problems such as untreated cavities or gingivitis, visit your dentist before using any home teeth-whitening product. When it comes to whitening your teeth, you must take extra care if you have dental problems. Consult

your dentist, who can offer the safest course of treatment and provide further guidance.

89. Use a tooth-whitening toothpaste, but don't expect miracles on badly discolored teeth. Tooth whitening toothpaste does not bleach teeth, so it can't remove existing stains. But it does help remove much of the plaque on your teeth, and can remove staining chemicals before they have a chance to discolor those pearly whites.

90. See your doctor before taking any steps toward whitening your teeth with store-bought products. It might be that you simply need a professional cleaning. Your dentist can tell you if your gums are healthy. If you have any inflammation it is wise to wait on the whitening treatment until your gums are in better condition.

91. To keep water from staining your teeth, avoid fluoride. While fluoride can be good for your teeth's overall health, many people have reported that it leaves their teeth discolored. If there's fluoride in the tap water in your home, try installing a water purifier to minimize its effects on your teeth.

92. To whiten your teeth while you eat, use orange peels! Citrus fruits have great natural whitening

properties. Just take the peel from the orange and rub it across your teeth after you finish eating. Let it sit for a few minutes, and then brush your teeth like you normally would. You should see the results right away.

93. To make your teeth look their best after a bleaching session, be sure to focus on your gums. Red or irritated gums will distract from your teeth, and may make them look less healthy than they actually are. Try using a gum massager before you have your teeth whitened. It'll make sure part of your smile looks great.

94. When you are trying to get a whiter smile, you should try brushing your teeth with teeth whitening toothpastes. These toothpastes can remove mild discoloration on your teeth through subtle abrasives that they contain. Get the smile that you have always wanted when you begin brushing your teeth with teeth whitening toothpaste.

95. Make sure to contact your dentist before starting to use an over the counter tooth whitening treatment. No one wants to wait for whiter teeth, but discoloration could be a sign of a more serious issue. Take the time to let your doctor rule out any issues and then whiten away.

96. Using whitening toothpaste is a common strategy. While they will not have the same effect as a tooth whitening procedure, they are great as a maintenance tool to stop new stains forming. By using an abrasive, your toothpaste will scrub the stains off without harming your enamel.

97. Avoid wearing shirts that are bright white if you want to hide a less than perfect smile. The white shade will only make any stains on your teeth even more obvious. Choose off white or cream colors that will help avoid your stains looking worse. Smile big in the morning after you've gotten dressed to see if your outfit is hurting you.

98. Don't believe that a toothpaste can whiten your teeth. The toothpaste may perform this action to a certain degree, but you will have to use multiple methods as well if you wish to clear away discoloration. If you do buy a toothpaste that promises to whiten your teeth, make sure it contains baking soda.

99. Consult your dentist and see if she sells a home teeth-whitening gel for use after you have left the office. Using this method, your dentist will give you a mouth piece that you wear, filled with a

whitening gel. Using this method can make your teeth several shades whiter.

100.   One important teeth whitening tip is to try to always brush and floss your teeth even when not at home. This is important to prevent the build up of plaque. Bring a toothbrush and floss with you at work and also when you go out to eat. At the very least, try to wash your mouth out after a meal.

101.   Laser tooth whitening is an effective procedure that can produce quick results. This procedure is probably the quickest solution when you want your teeth whitened and brightened. After a bleaching agent is applied to the teeth, a laser is used to activate the whitening properties. Your teeth will look much whiter than before, by up to five magnitudes.

102.   Floss daily. Flossing daily will help you keep up with other proper dental hygiene habits. Flossing and brushing are imperative to having clean, white teeth. Carry a spare toothbrush and floss with you in your glove box, bag, or purse so that you can brush if you are going to be away from your house.

103.   Approximately half of all patients who try some sort of whitening treatment, especially those at home, will experience some level of tooth sensitivity as a result. If this happens to you, try lowering the concentration of the product that you are using, and see if that corrects the problem.

104.   Use natural tooth whiteners, such as baking soda, orange peels, or lemon peels. Mixing any of these with a little salt can make an excellent cheap tooth whitening product. Be sure to wash your mouth out thoroughly after using any of these methods, as the harsh acids can damage your teeth.

105.   Try natural remedies to whiten your teeth. Hydrogen peroxide and baking soda have long been known to whiten teeth. These can be used together as a paste to brush your teeth with. You can also swish with a mixture of peroxide and water two or three times daily. This will not only whiten your teeth but will improve the overall state of your oral health.

106.   Once you eliminate the stains on your teeth with a teeth whitening treatment, you do not have to repeat the process too often. Really if you do not consume a lot of coffee, smoke or

drink large amounts of wine, you may only have to touch up the whiteness as little as once a year.

107.   To keep water from staining your teeth, avoid fluoride. While fluoride can be good for your teeth's overall health, many people have reported that it leaves their teeth discolored. If there's fluoride in the tap water in your home, try installing a water purifier to minimize its effects on your teeth.

108.   To get better results from any natural teeth whitening method, add a little white vinegar! Vinegar is a great way to make baking soda, lemon juice, and other household whitening methods more effective. The vinegar works as a sort of primer for your teeth that will help any whitener to sink in and have a stronger effect.

109.   To keep your teeth white, be sure to use a straw when you are drinking beverages with high levels of acidity. The acidity in beverages, like sodas or sports drinks, can affect the color of your teeth, but the straw acts as a barrier. This will not change the color of your teeth overnight and if your teeth are already stained it will not take off the stain. It will help to prevent more discoloration.

110.   Eat fibrous produce. It cleans your teeth naturally and is a healthy snack. Several examples that are good scrubbers are apples, cucumbers, broccoli and carrots. You should eat them raw, then chew them up really well so you allow time for the teeth to be worked on. Chew on both sides of your mouth so that all of your teeth will be cleaned.

111.   If you are looking to get whiter teeth, you should not smoke. The nicotine content in cigarettes causes your teeth to stain a dark color. If you really want to get a bright white smile, then you need to make sure that you quit smoking for good, so that your teeth do not redevelop a stain.

112.   Change your diet for whiter teeth. Avoid processed foods and foods high in sugar. Replace them with lots of raw fruits and vegetables that help clean your teeth while you eat them and promote healthy salivation during chewing. Not only will this help whiten you teeth, it will also keep them strong and healthy.

113.   For whiter teeth at home, try doing a baking soda brushing once a week. This helps remove stains and it helps whiten your teeth. Brush like you would with toothpaste, but you replace the

toothpaste with the baking soda. You can use it as an alternative to toothpaste too. If it irritates gums, try using salt.

114.   Prevention of staining is one way to keep your teeth whiter. Some of the things you drink can cause discoloration of your teeth. Coffee, tea, wine and soda are all notorious for causing stains on teeth. If you will sip them or drink them through a straw this will help them to not make as much contact with your teeth. Also, when you are done with your drink, rinse your mouth with water.

115.   One important teeth whitening tip is to make sure that you always drink plenty of water. This will act as a natural way to remove extra food and harmful materials from your teeth, keeping them whiter. Be sure to rinse with water after eating as often as possible.

116.   If you use mouthwash, stay away from the green and blue colors that contain alcohol. The alcohol will dry out the surface of your teeth and make them prone to discoloration. Look for mouthwashes that do not contain alcohol or cut down on your overall usage of mouthwash.

117.   If you want to whiten your teeth naturally, then look no further that your box of baking soda. This is one of the most proven home remedies. Make a paste with baking soda and water and brush your teeth using this paste, and then rinse. When done consistently, you will soon have gleaming white teeth.

118.   Rinse out your mouth with one percent hydrogen peroxide. Hydrogen peroxide strips are expensive to buy and harsh on your teeth. Keep the peroxide in your mouth for at least a minute and make sure you do not swallow an excessive amount of the solution. Follow up by brushing your teeth.

119.   Use natural tooth whiteners, such as baking soda, orange peels, or lemon peels. Mixing any of these with a little salt can make an excellent cheap tooth whitening product. Be sure to wash your mouth out thoroughly after using any of these methods, as the harsh acids can damage your teeth.

120.   Rinse your mouth with hydrogen peroxide before you brush your teeth. This is a natural remedy that is cheap and works well. It will help whiten your teeth and it isn't as harsh as other

whitening methods. Be careful not to swallow it because it will make you sick and possibly vomit.

121.   Try natural remedies to whiten your teeth. Hydrogen peroxide and baking soda have long been known to whiten teeth. These can be used together as a paste to brush your teeth with. You can also swish with a mixture of peroxide and water two or three times daily. This will not only whiten your teeth but will improve the overall state of your oral health.

122.   To whiten teeth, try brushing with baking soda. Baking soda naturally whitens teeth and serves as a natural remedy for discolored teeth. When using baking soda to whiten your teeth, brush gently to avoid irritating your gums.

123.   To keep water from staining your teeth, avoid fluoride. While fluoride can be good for your teeth's overall health, many people have reported that it leaves their teeth discolored. If there's fluoride in the tap water in your home, try installing a water purifier to minimize its effects on your teeth.

124.   Practice good oral hygiene to whiten your teeth and keep your smile bright. Brush your teeth at least twice a day and floss regularly to

remove food particles that become trapped between them. Taking good care of your teeth is one of the best ways to keep them clean, white and healthy for years to come.

125.   For the most effective at-home teeth whitening, call a few local dentists' offices and ask for the name brand of the whitening products they use in their office or what they send home with patients to use. Most often, all of those products are readily available online for a much less expensive price than through your dental care provider.

126.   To get professional teeth whitening done at an affordable price, look for a dental school or dental hygiene training program in your area and let a student dentist or hygienist do the job. Costs at dental schools are much, much less than at a professional dental office and while the work is carried out by a student, there is always a licensed dentist on-hand supervising all work done by the students.

127.   Stop whitening your teeth if the treatment causes pain or sensitivity. Teeth whitening products can often lead to increased sensitivity and could result in inflammation. If any of these problems occur, discontinue your use of the

product immediately, and make an appointment with your dentist to talk about other options.

128.   Apply a sunless tanner to make your teeth appear whiter. The color you will get from applying a tanner provides a contrast to your teeth that will make them gleam whiter than when you are paler. As an added benefit, it will also make your eyes stand out even more.

129.   To whiten your teeth, you can buy whitening strips from any drug store. Not only are these strips inexpensive, but they are said to help whiten your teeth by 2 or 3 shades. Be sure that these whitening strips around a 4 percent peroxide solution for the most effective results.

130.   A great teeth whitening tip is to avoid smoking. Smoking is one of the worst things you can do if you are trying to keep your teeth white. The nicotine in cigarettes will cause them to turn a yellowish hue that is very hard or impossible to reverse.

131.   A great way to naturally whiten your teeth without resorting to harsh chemicals is to use a lemon juice and salt mixture. Using this mixture as a mouthwash is a cheap and effective way that

way to remove surface stains from your teeth. Be sure to rinse with water afterward.

132.   Use the peel off an orange to whiten your teeth. You can rub an orange peel on your teeth to make them whiter. Alternatively, you can even grind up some of the orange peel. Combine this with bay leaves and form it into a paste. Brush this paste onto your teeth then rinse.

133.   Quit smoking if you want whiter teeth. Smoking destroys the enamel on your teeth. What is left behind is brown or yellow teeth. Even if you pay for an expensive dental whitening, your smile won't gleam for long if you smoke. Quit smoking for your health, but also for your appearance. You'll be happy that you did.

134.   Going to a dentist and paying to have your teeth bleached is very effective. Bleaching solution is applied to the teeth and it stays there for about an hour. Do not worry about taste or burns because they take precautions to prevent this from happening to you. Results can usually be seen after just one session.

135.   You can make an appointment with your dentist, and have them perform laser teeth

whitening. This will be the best way to get make teeth as white as they can be. The dentist applies a gel, and then the bleaching agents in the gel are activated with the laser. Your teeth are instantly whiter than before by 5-6 times.

136.   Use natural tooth whiteners, such as baking soda, orange peels, or lemon peels. Mixing any of these with a little salt can make an excellent cheap tooth whitening product. Be sure to wash your mouth out thoroughly after using any of these methods, as the harsh acids can damage your teeth.

137.   Be sure that the teeth whitening trays fit your mouth correctly. If they do not fit well there is a good chance that they are going to cause you problems with your gums. If you notice that your gums are more sensitive or in any pain, stop using the product and see your dentist.

138.   Increase the amount of foods in your diet that clean your teeth. These include high-fiber fruits and vegetables such as carrots, apples, celery, and cauliflower. These work to whiten your teeth by scrubbing off plaque as you eat. They also cause your mouth to produce more saliva, which results in healthier enamel and whiter teeth.

139.   One of the fastest ways to get pearly white teeth is by using an electric toothbrush. These toothbrushes are highly recommended by many dentists because they eliminate more plaque than regular toothbrushes. Other benefits of using an electric toothbrush include better protection from cavities and gingivitis.

140.   Use whitening strips. Depending on how badly your teeth are stained, they usually don't immediately work. Over time, you will notice your teeth getting whiter. You should use these strips regularly, but not too much. These strips are easy and convenient to use and keep you from visiting the dentist.

141.   If you use a tray to whiten your teeth, be sure it fits on your teeth. If the tray does fit right, it can cause problems with your gums. If this happens stop using the product as soon as you find out.

142.   Strawberries, among other fruits, work as excellent teeth whiteners. Eat them regularly and make sure to bite into them with your front teeth to reap the benefits of their teeth-whitening properties. Another way to utilize strawberries to whiten teeth is to mash them in a paste, apply

and leave on for 5 minutes. Make sure to rinse thoroughly afterward to remove the sugars.

143.   For the whitest and cleanest teeth possible, invest in an effective electric tooth brush. The more expensive models of electric toothbrushes can help brush your teeth more effectively than humanly possible with a manual toothbrush. Make sure you invest in a rechargeable electric toothbrush with replaceable heads for the best value.

144.   Keep your expectations realistic when you whiten your teeth, whatever method you use. If your expectations are out of touch with reality, you won't be satisfied with the results. There are many different factors that can effect the teeth whitening process. One being your age, and the second being what your teeth looked like before you start whitening. Talk to a dentist before trying to whiten your teeth so that you are aware of what to expect.

145.   It is a common myth that lemon or lime juice can whiten your teeth. In fact, the recommendation is to stay far away from each of them. Lemon and limes have acids that can erode enamel and cause your teeth to be more discolored.

146.   As a woman, the selection you make in terms of your lipstick or lipgloss instantly affects the shade of your teeth. One of the most versatile and neutral shades to making your teeth appear whiter are nude pinks with a brownish undertone. This will even out your complexion, finish your look, and make your teeth look great,too!

147.   An easy way to make your eyes and teeth look instantly whiter is to make use of a self-tanning product that you can apply at home or a spray tan you can have done in a salon. The darker your skin, the more apparent the white in your teeth and eyes will be.

148.   You need to use a toothpaste with a whitening agent, and baking soda is a great additive to look for as well. Any brand will do, but Arm & Hammer is one of the best toothpastes. It is also suggested that you brush twice or more a day in order to create a teeth whitening experience.

149.   Use baking soda to whiten your smile. You can either purchase toothpaste that has baking soda included, or you can create your own whitener. To do this, combine baking soda with

salt and brush your teeth with the mixture. Try to do this at least once per day to get the maximum benefit from your home remedy technique.

150.   Before you whiten your teeth, talk to your dentist about which product to use. There are many different teeth whitening products for you to choose from. Oftentimes, these products can be expensive and even damaging so it's important that you chose the right one. To avoid most of the hassle just ask your dentist. They generally have good advice when it comes to teeth whitening.

151.   Be careful using "home remedies" to whiten your teeth. Common home remedies like lemons, ash, or baking soda can actually do more damage than good. You should ask your dentist for "home remedy" suggestions if you cannot afford a professional procedure.

152.   When you are going through a teeth whitening process, you may experience sensitivity. Sensitivity during the whitening is very common. The sensitivity should disappear within a day or two after the process is over. If you have continued sensitivity, you should

consult with your dentist about the problem that you are having.

153.   Use a straw when drinking highly acidic beverages, such as sodas or citrus juices. Using a straw will help divert the acid away from your teeth, into your mouth, which can keep it from causing damage to your teeth. Gray teeth are often caused by thinning tooth enamel, so protecting your tooth enamel will keep your teeth whiter.

154.   Rinse your mouth out after drinking coffee or tea. They are both well known for staining teeth. For better results, try to eliminate it from your diet altogether. The same goes for soda and wine; they can stain your teeth just as much, if not more than coffee and tea.

155.   If you are looking to whiten your teeth then you may want to consider avoiding some bad habits which can cause tooth discoloration. The three big culprits are coffee, soda, and cigarettes. By avoiding these there things you will make it so much easier to whiten your teeth and keep them that way.

156.   To whiten your teeth while you eat, use orange peels! Citrus fruits have great natural

whitening properties. Just take the peel from the orange and rub it across your teeth after you finish eating. Let it sit for a few minutes, and then brush your teeth like you normally would. You should see the results right away.

157.	When trying to whiten your teeth, use toothpaste specifically made for teeth whitening. These toothpastes use peroxides that act as a bleaching agent for your teeth. Be sure to look at the amount of peroxide in the toothpaste, typically the concentration is between ten and twenty percent. Choose a product in the middle, and if your teeth tolerate the toothpaste (and you want more effective whitening), move up to a toothpaste with 20% peroxide.

158.	Consume an adequate amount of calcium each day to make teeth stronger. Some studies have been done which indicate that cheese can start to rebuild tooth enamel due to the calcium in it. Keeping your enamel healthy means your teeth will be beautiful and white, so snack on cheese several times a week.

159.	There are a variety of home ingredients that you can use to get your smile looking a little whiter. You can try using lemon juice or baking soda to help get a cleaner smile. Many home ingredients have been proven to give you a whiter smile with little effort.

160.   One method of whitening your teeth is by brushing with the juice from strawberries. The acid causes the tooth enamel to soften, allowing you to easily remove stains. Compared with other methods, this approach is very affordable.

161.   One of the primary causes of having discolored teeth and smile in general is bad habits with beverages. Coffee is one of the leading causes of having teeth that are discolored. If you are determined to continue drinking coffee then you will want to brush your teeth immediately after each cup.

162.   The first line of defense against any type of discoloring problem is a dental regimen that includes a whitening toothpaste as well as a mouthwash to help with this. While these things alone won't be able to completely whiten your teeth they will be a very good start to give you a good base.

163.   When you decide to do any kind of dental regimen that includes whitening your teeth you should be sure to have the advice of a dental professional. If you try to do things completely

on your own you may make amateur mistakes that will set back your progress by several months.

164.   Since most teeth whitening gels are so powerful, only a dentist can give them to you. Teeth whitening gel is used in conjunction with laser whitening and only the laser equipment will activate it. This is a more costly method than others, but lasts longer and works quicker.

165.   Use a mixture of hydrogen peroxide and water to make a rinse to whiten your teeth. Not only does hydrogen peroxide kill germs, it also acts as a whitening agent. Many companies make a "whitening" mouthwash with water, hydrogen peroxide and mint flavor. Save money by making your own rinse.

166.   It may be necessary for you to drink less coffee or go without it altogether if you want whiter teeth. Coffee is one of the main reasons for stained and yellow teeth. By drinking it on a regular basis, you're adding to the problem. While cutting out coffee can be difficult, it's definitely worth it. Treat yourself to a steaming cup of hot chocolate instead.

167.   Before you commit to a certain over-the-counter teeth whitener, you may want to check online reviews or ask your friends for their experience with it. Many times, people pay ridiculous amounts for a product that promises to whiten their teeth, when in reality, it does absolutely nothing to help or makes teeth color worse.

168.   You should keep in mind that teeth whitening only works for your real, natural teeth. It will not work on any crowns, veneers, implants, or fillings you have in your mouth. So if you have a lot of these, it may not be worth the expense of trying to whiten your teeth.

169.   To avoid unnecessary pain, people with sensitive teeth should consult a dental professional to find the best possible whitening product. Since most take home teeth whitening products are not made for sensitive teeth, it is important that you consult a professional before applying an irritant to your own sensitive teeth. They can direct you to the most effective and pain-free whitening solution.

170.   To have a white smile, make sure you avoid drinking water or using toothpastes that contain fluoride. It has been reported that fluoride may

aid in discoloring and permanently staining your teeth. Many countries have actually banned fluoride from their drinking water due to this very reason. To stay on the safe side, avoid fluoride at all costs for a healthy and white smile.

171.	You may not be able to brush after every meal, however, you can rinse your mouth after meals. Take a minute or two after eating or drinking beverages that can stain and thoroughly rinse your mouth. This will help remove loose particles and stain causing residues that may be left behind from your meals.

172.	Brush with magnesium oil for whiter teeth. Magnesium oil is a brine made from magnesium chloride and water. It is called an oil because the resulting mixture has an oily appearance and texture. Adding a couple of drops to your toothbrush when brushing, or swishing with a few drops mixed with water, can make your teeth significantly whiter.

173.	Whitening toothpaste is one of the simplest remedies for whiter teeth. Whitening toothpaste removes stains while also helping to remove plaque. Your teeth will have the stains removed and will appear brighter eventually.

174. If you are looking for an easy way to get a whiter, brighter smile, then you should try using teeth whitening strips. These strips are a convenient way to get your smile looking great because they are so easy to use. These strips contain peroxide, which help to clean the outside of your teeth.

175. Use whitening strips. Depending on how badly your teeth are stained, they usually don't immediately work. Over time, you will notice your teeth getting whiter. You should use these strips regularly, but not too much. These strips are easy and convenient to use and keep you from visiting the dentist.

176. If your teeth are heavily strained or if over-the-counter products have failed to work, you may want to visit a dentist to receive a professional cleaning. While this method carries a heftier price tag than other solutions, it produces faster, immediate results.

177. Most smokers already know that smoking leaves their teeth dull looking and discolored. Smokers will always have a much harder time in whitening their teeth than non-smokers. Stopping smoking will improve the color of your

teeth drastically. Not to mention, not smoking is just better for your health.

178.   Before undertaking any at-home whitening projects, consult with your dentist about your teeth. If you have any issues with gums or cavities, whitening methods bought over the counter can have a negative impact on your mouth. Tell your dentist what you want to try and ask for a green light before you proceed.

179.   If you feel any discomfort in your mouth or teeth, stop your teeth whitening regimen at home. Using certain whitening products can increase sensitivity and inflammation. If pain or other uncomfortable sensations arise, do not use at-home whitening products until you consult with your dentist. He or she may have suggestions for alternate procedures that will be more comfortable.

180.   Use the right shade of lipstick and lip gloss to brighten your teeth. If your teeth are yellowing or off white, go with nudes and pinks with blue undertones. If you have graying teeth, a cool tone with a brown base will do the trick in making your teeth pop.

181.   To whiten your teeth, you can buy whitening strips from any drug store. Not only are these strips inexpensive, but they are said to help whiten your teeth by 2 or 3 shades. Be sure that these whitening strips around a 4 percent peroxide solution for the most effective results.

182.   If you are going to the dentist to have bleaching treatments, be sure not to overdo it. People get excited at the results they see, so they think their teeth will get even whiter if they continuously get them bleached. Unfortunately, the only result of this are teeth that turn blue!

183.   Brush your teeth as soon as you wake up, and as soon as you want to go to bed to see your teeth get whiter. As you sleep, your mouth dries out and creates plaque as bacteria builds up.

184.   Use whitening toothpaste. Any kind of toothpaste is a whitener but a toothpaste with a whitening agent in it will speed up the process. Regular flossing of your teeth will also prevent stains from plaque before they occur. Both will help keep your teeth whiter for a longer time period.

185.   Peroxide is one of the most popular home remedies for whitening teeth. To use peroxide,

brush your teeth like normal, and then swish with peroxide afterward. Another way to use peroxide is to dip a cotton ball in the peroxide and rub it on your teeth. You should see results in a couple weeks.

186.   To avoid unnecessary pain, people with sensitive teeth should consult a dental professional to find the best possible whitening product. Since most take home teeth whitening products are not made for sensitive teeth, it is important that you consult a professional before applying an irritant to your own sensitive teeth. They can direct you to the most effective and pain-free whitening solution.

187.   If you over use teeth whitening products, especially extremely powerful ones, you could be doing serious harm to your teeth. You should always consult with your dentist before going through such a procedure and make sure it's safe for you to do so. If your dentist says it's too soon or you've done it too many times - listen to him!

188.   Eating a diet with plenty of whole and raw foods is great for your teeth. Vegetables are great for helping clean your teeth. They also do not contain harsh processed ingredients that may

stick to your teeth and cause unwanted tooth decay and discolorations.

189.   Determine why your teeth are discolored before starting any whitening treatment. A trip to your dentist should answer this question. Knowing the cause of your discolored teeth will give you the best treatment options for your specific problems and therefore you will also get the best results too.

190.   Save your orange peel and have a teeth whitening session. The inside of the orange peel has citric acid and can help to remove stains and whiten teeth. Either rub it directly on your teeth or get some dried peel, organically grown and some ground up bay leaves to create a paste that you can brush on. Remember to brush after your session to remove any acid that may harm the enamel over time.

191.   Your eating habits are a big key to maintaining a white smile. Processed food and fast food contain chemicals and preservatives that can leave staining residues on your teeth. Try to incorporate fresh raw vegetables and fruits and eat salads which contain beneficial vitamins and minerals that help promote stronger, healthier teeth.

192.   Beverages that contain acid or carbonation are best drunk with a straw to help keep your teeth white. By using a straw you can divert the beverages past the teeth and prevent some of the staining potential. Try not to fill your mouth with beverage when drinking as this will defeat the purpose of the straw.

193.   A great way to whiten your teeth is to use tooth whitening strips. Usually you will use these once or twice a day to both the top and the bottom. Leave it on for the appointed time then take it off. In a few weeks you should be a few shades whiter.

194.   Pay close attention to the state of your mouth when using at-home teeth whitening products. For some people these treatments can cause temporary, mild tooth sensitivity. If you are using a product with a tray that does not fit your mouth well this can irritate your gums. Discontinue the treatments if you experience discomfort or pain.

195.   Use dried, crushed holy basil leaves to whiten your teeth. This is a known method for naturally whitening your teeth and is very effective. It is also very good for your keeping

your gums healthy. This is a great way to whiten your teeth and has positive oral health benefits.

196.   The chemicals that are used to help whiten your teeth can cause your gums and other soft tissues in your mouth to become irritated. These caustic chemicals can make your mouth feel like it is in a whole world of hurt. Make sure you talk to your doctor about any problems that you experience.

197.   A professional whitening may be expensive, but it's probably the best way to start whitening your teeth. The procedure provided by your dentist has immediate results but can be more costly than the do it yourself products.

198.   If you have opted for a teeth whitening treatment, you should keep your teeth free of food particles by brushing whenever you've eaten. This is because bacteria will grow on the teeth due to the food remnants. Following most whitening treatments, your teeth are especially vulnerable to this bacteria, so you have to be scrupulous about brushing.

199.   A natural way to help whiten your teeth is to eat fruits and vegetables that are fibrous in texture. These types of foods act as a natural

cleanser, scrubbing the teeth while you are eating them. Some great choices for fibrous fruits and vegetables are apples, cucumber, carrots and broccoli.

200.   People who are fans of red wines, especially ones who have been drinking it forever, are more likely to have discolored teeth. Red wine has a deep red color that gets absorbed by tooth enamel and is difficult to remove with normal brushing. The only way to resolve this issue is to cut back on the amount of red wine you drink.

201.   To make your teeth look whiter via makeup, wear red lipstick! Deep reds and other blue based colors create a visual illusion of whiter teeth. By the same token, you should avoid any warmer colors like yellows or browns. The colors will create an effect that highlights the yellowest parts of your teeth.

202.   It is important that you brush and floss your teeth, as well as message your gums twice every day. The best way in which to maintain white teeth is to brush and floss after eating. This way, you are going to be sure to remove the plaque and the food that build up and cause stains on your teeth.

203.   Some whitening strips can cause damage to your gums. Avoid products that require you to leave them on for hours. The whitening process will take longer to work than with the two-hour strips, but the increase in gum sensitivity associated with the two-hour treatment is much more likely to appear.

204.   If you have gum disease or untreated cavities in your mouth, be cautious before undergoing any teeth whitening procedures. You could end up damaging your teeth even further or just end up wasting money on a procedure that won't work. You should consult with your dentist before undergoing the procedure.

205.   To maintain white teeth, you should have regular professional cleanings done. Get your teeth cleaned by your dentist every six month and adopt good habits at home too. Though it is common to procrastinate on doing this, take advantage of the fact that most dental plans cover two cleanings per year.

206.   Strawberries are one food that can naturally whiten your teeth. The natural compounds contained within strawberries will whiten your teeth and eliminate the need to expose them to chemicals. You can utilize the strawberry in one

of two ways; cut it into two and rub over the teeth while indulging in your favorite at home activity, or turn the strawberry into a mashed paste and leave this to sit on your teeth for five minutes.

207.   The first step in obtaining the pearliest whites you can imagine is simply to brush your teeth every day, two times per day. It may seem obvious, but many people put all of their faith in tooth whitening products when simply brushing your teeth often is usually the first and best course of action.

208.   Use dried, crushed holy basil leaves to whiten your teeth. This is a known method for naturally whitening your teeth and is very effective. It is also very good for your keeping your gums healthy. This is a great way to whiten your teeth and has positive oral health benefits.

209.   When trying to whiten your teeth, use toothpaste specifically made for teeth whitening. These toothpastes use peroxides that act as a bleaching agent for your teeth. Be sure to look at the amount of peroxide in the toothpaste, typically the concentration is between ten and twenty percent. Choose a product in the middle, and if your teeth tolerate the toothpaste (and you

want more effective whitening), move up to a toothpaste with 20% peroxide.

210.   If you are trying to get your teeth as white as you can try using a whitening toothpaste a few times a day. This toothpaste works great at getting rid of stains on your teeth. Over time, the stains will dissipate and your teeth will become brighter.

211.   To maintain the results of your whitening, stay away from cigarettes and processed foods. Teeth friendly foods like apples, celery, and carrots will keep your teeth healthy and bright. Chewing on a sugar free gum can also be very helpful, as it stimulates the production of saliva, which can lead to a cleaner mouth.

212.   Schedule regular appointments to have your teeth cleaned. Yearly appointments for teeth cleanings are recommended. Many people do who do not visit the dentist on a regular basis are quick to buy harsh chemicals to whiten their teeth later. Avoid stained teeth and harsh chemicals completely by having your teeth cleaned at the dentist at least once a year.

213.   Consider using Vaseline as a means of whitening your teeth. While the taste will not be

entirely pleasant, the barrier created by the Vaseline will protect your teeth.

214.   Baking soda is great for whitening teeth, plus, it is inexpensive and easy to get. Purchase tooth paste with baking soda in it for extra whitening every day. You can also make your own whitening paste by mixing baking soda with a pinch of salt. Rub this paste on your teeth, let it sit for a few minutes and then brush as usual.

215.   Brush and floss at least a twice a day. This will help to prevent a buildup of plaque, which can discolor your teeth. It is also a good idea to carry floss with you, that way you can floss anytime after you eat. Paying special attention to your teeth will help to prevent staining.

216.   A great way to naturally whiten your teeth without resorting to harsh chemicals is to use a baking soda and salt mixture. This is a method that has been used by many people for a long time, that is both safe and cost effective. There are plenty of toothpaste products that use baking soda in them.

217.   If you are willing to go to any length to get your teeth whitened, go to your dentist. Dentists can use specialized equipment, along with the

bleaching chemicals, to whiten your smile around 15 shades in one session. The cost of professional teeth whitening is around 500 dollars each time.

218.   Use hydrogen peroxide as a mouth rinse to whiten your teeth without using harsh chemicals. Hydrogen peroxide is gentler on tooth enamel than commercial whitening strips and can whiten your teeth significantly if used regularly. Do not swallow the liquid, and brush your teeth immediately after rinsing with hydrogen peroxide.

219.   Reduce or eliminate consumption of beverages that typically stain teeth in order to brighten your smile. Beverages such as coffee, tea or red wine can stain teeth, especially if the liquid stays on the teeth for some time. Either brush soon after drinking these beverages or use a straw to reduce staining and discoloration.

220.   To avoid unnecessary pain, people with sensitive teeth should consult a dental professional to find the best possible whitening product. Since most take home teeth whitening products are not made for sensitive teeth, it is important that you consult a professional before applying an irritant to your own sensitive teeth.

They can direct you to the most effective and pain-free whitening solution.

221.   Cut back on beverages that are known to have a staining effect on your teeth. Red wine and coffee are some of the worse known culprits of putting stains on your pearly whites. If you cannot avoid them all together try drinking them thorough a straw. The liquid will have less contact with your teeth.

222.   Keep regular teeth cleaning appointments with your dentist. They are necessary appointments, that make your smile brighter which results in more confidence. These should be done one to two times a year, especially if you're a smoker.

223.   Try not to drink water that contains fluoride or using any toothpaste that contains it. Contrary to the popular belief that it is good for your teeth it has been shown to have a staining effect! Other countries have all together banned the use of it in their water because of dangers.

224.   Be careful with excessive whitening of your teeth. If you have repeatedly whitened your teeth, you may be causing irreparable damage to the teeth. You should avoid using powerful

whitening products repeatedly. If you are not receiving the results from the whitening, consult your dentist to find other ways to whiten.

225.   After you have used a teeth whitening program, do not use a mouth wash with alcohol in it. The alcohol can actually diminish the effects of the program and revert your results or dramatically lower them. On the other side, an oxyegenating mouth wash may actually benefit the teeth whitening regimen.

226.   When you are whitening your teeth, remember that there are limitations to what it can do. If you have had extensive dental treatments like caps, bridges or crowns, these will not be whitened by the treatment that you are using. You will have to have this work replaced to match your new whiter smile.

227.   Use a tooth-whitening toothpaste, but don't expect miracles on badly discolored teeth. Tooth whitening toothpaste does not bleach teeth, so it can't remove existing stains. But it does help remove much of the plaque on your teeth, and can remove staining chemicals before they have a chance to discolor those pearly whites.

228.   To get better looking teeth through your diet, eat more raw foods. Chewing raw foods can be great for your teeth, and avoiding processed foods means you'll develop less plaque. While raw foods aren't a good way to get quick teeth whitening results, eating them regularly will make your teeth sparkle over time.

229.   Whitening toothpaste can really help whiten your teeth. Stains will be removed when you use a whitening toothpaste by the rubbing. By brushing your teeth over time, stains are removed and your teeth will become whiter and brighter.

230.   One of the fastest ways to get pearly white teeth is by using an electric toothbrush. These toothbrushes are highly recommended by many dentists because they eliminate more plaque than regular toothbrushes. Other benefits of using an electric toothbrush include better protection from cavities and gingivitis.

231.   Visit your dentist twice a year. You should visit your dentist for a regular cleaning and checkup. Most people don't like going to the dentist but it's important to have healthy teeth and will help with keeping your teeth white.

Keep your appointments with your dentist and visit them regularly.

232.　If your teeth need quite a bit of whitening, you may want to consider consulting a dentist. While certainly more expensive, whitening done by a professional is much quicker than any other methods.

233.　For whiter teeth, stay away from white wines. White wines generally contain more acid than red wines, which will eat away at the enamel of your teeth.

234.　Strawberries, among other fruits, work as excellent teeth whiteners. Eat them regularly and make sure to bite into them with your front teeth to reap the benefits of their teeth-whitening properties. Another way to utilize strawberries to whiten teeth is to mash them in a paste, apply and leave on for 5 minutes. Make sure to rinse thoroughly afterward to remove the sugars.

235.　An electric toothbrush is an excellent investment if you are trying to whiten your teeth. This helps to remove teeth stains caused by certain foods, wine and tobacco. They remove any yellowness that may be embedded in the surface of your teeth.

236.   Believe it or not, you can use sage to get your teeth whiter. Not only is this safe because you are using a natural product, but it has been proven to be very effective. All you have to do is buy sage leaves and rub them in a circular motion onto your teeth.

237.   A great way to gradually whiten discolored teeth is by using a whitening toothpaste. Whitening toothpastes have proven very effective at whitening teeth. Using a quality whitening toothpaste is one of the cheapest ways to get your teeth white. There are many choices on the market for whitening toothpastes.

238.   One important teeth whitening tip is to try to consume as many raw foods as possible when you are snacking or for your meal time. The reason for this is that these types of foods will act as natural ways to scrub your teeth and keep them looking as white as possible.

239.   An easy way to keep teeth whitened is to brush after consuming something that tends to stain teeth. Common culprits are coffee, sodas, wines, teas, berries, and sweets. If you brush immediately after consuming these items, you prevent the stain from setting into your teeth.

This will help you to keep your teeth white without having to resort to expensive treatments.

240.   Hydrogen peroxide is another alternative that you can use to brush your teeth. The peroxide oxidizes your teeth upon contact and can remove states. Most hydrogen peroxide you buy in stores will already be diluted, but you can dilute further, by mixing 2 tablespoons of water to every tablespoon of hydrogen peroxide. If you do not like the taste of the peroxide, substitute a sweet tasting mouthwash for the water.

241.   When you want whiter teeth, do not be fooled by the different kinds of toothpastes available. Toothpaste that claims to whiten your teeth is frequently more expensive than normal toothpaste. When trying to remove stains from your teeth, regular toothpaste works just as well and is often cheaper than whitening toothpaste.

242.   Using a home whitening remedy may not be the best idea when trying to whiten your teeth. If you are thinking about using home products, such as lemon, ash, or baking soda, you may want to reconsider. Using these home remedies can damage your teeth in the long run.

243.   It is important to include raw fruits and vegetables in your diet, to help keep your teeth strong and healthy. Fatty foods increase the chance of cavities and can cause discoloration of your teeth. Try to stay away from these kinds of foods when at all possible to help your teeth remain healthy. Snacking throughout the day can also dull or discolor your teeth.

244.   Ask your dentist about the different teeth whitening options available to you. Some dentists may recommend a procedure that they provide in their office. Some may refer you to a certain product that you can find at your local pharmacy. Some may simply suggest that you brush your teeth more often.

245.   Use natural tooth whiteners, such as baking soda, orange peels, or lemon peels. Mixing any of these with a little salt can make an excellent cheap tooth whitening product. Be sure to wash your mouth out thoroughly after using any of these methods, as the harsh acids can damage your teeth.

246.   Keep a toothbrush on hand so you can brush after eating sticky or sugary snacks. Sugary foods can stick to teeth, and start staining them very quickly. Right after finishing your snack, use

your mini-toothbrush to clean your teeth for a minute or two. Even without toothpaste, giving your teeth a good scrub and rinsing thoroughly with water will prevent food stains from setting.

247.   Mix baking soda and salt together for an at-home whitening method. This is a well known treatment for making teeth whiter. You can make a paste out of it by mixing them together with a little bit of water. Make sure you rinse your mouth out well afterwards.

248.   In order to get white teeth a good habit that you can do is to choose to eat food that naturally whitens teeth. Examples of these are raw fruits and vegetables that scrub your teeth while you eat them. These foods include carrots, strawberries, apples, celery, pineapples, oranges and pears.

249.   To prevent your teeth from discoloring, you should always use a straw when drinking. The straw helps in reducing the time the beverage has to stain your teeth. It makes the liquid go straight down towards your throat, bypassing your teeth.

250.   Many people give up coffee and move to tea in an attempt to have whiter teeth. While this has not been proven to actually whiten teeth it will

certainly help to prevent further discoloring. This is because coffee is one of the worst things you can do to the color of your teeth.

251.   One important teeth whitening tip is to try to avoid beverages that will stain your teeth. There are many liquids that can cause damage that is hard to reverse. Drinks to avoid if possible are carrot juice, red wine, coffee, tea, and cola. If you do choose to dring any of these drinks, be sure to clean your teeth soon afterward.

252.   While you are brushing your teeth, you are protecting your teeth. You should use toothpaste specifically made to whiten teeth. There are many options, so do some research, and it will help you find the best whitening toothpaste for your needs.

253.   For the whitest and cleanest teeth possible, invest in an effective electric tooth brush. The more expensive models of electric toothbrushes can help brush your teeth more effectively than humanly possible with a manual toothbrush. Make sure you invest in a rechargeable electric toothbrush with replaceable heads for the best value.

254.   If you want to whiten your teeth, use whitening strips. Whitening strips are very popular and are a simple and quick way to whiten your teeth. Simply stick the strips to your teeth. Let them stay there for several minutes, and then take them off. Repeat this for several days until you get the whitening you desire.

255.   Before you commit to a certain over-the-counter teeth whitener, you may want to check online reviews or ask your friends for their experience with it. Many times, people pay ridiculous amounts for a product that promises to whiten their teeth, when in reality, it does absolutely nothing to help or makes teeth color worse.

256.   If you want a natural, great way to make your teeth whiter, try fresh lemons. Just rub a lemon peel's inner portion on your teeth each day to obtain teeth that look whiter and brighter. The approach to whiter teeth is very cost effective and can be applied quickly and simply. Lemon peels whiten teeth without having to use harsh chemicals, which are found in many of the whiteners on the market.

257.   Approximately half of all patients who try some sort of whitening treatment, especially

those at home, will experience some level of tooth sensitivity as a result. If this happens to you, try lowering the concentration of the product that you are using, and see if that corrects the problem.

258.   Make sure that you brush your teeth and floss daily after every meal. Flossing and brushing prevents the buildup of unwanted plaque which also discolors your teeth. Plaque is something you want to avoid at all costs and carrying floss with you can greatly help. Focusing on your teeth can assist in preventing discoloration and damage, keeping you healthy for the long term.

259.   Avoid drinking coffee, tea, cola, and wine unless you are drinking water with them or immediately afterward. These dark liquids have been shown to permanently stain and discolor teeth. Rinsing your mouth with water afterward can reduce these effects, as can brushing your teeth after your morning coffee, as it removes the staining chemicals from your mouth.

260.   Be sure that the teeth whitening trays fit your mouth correctly. If they do not fit well there is a good chance that they are going to cause you problems with your gums. If you notice that your

gums are more sensitive or in any pain, stop using the product and see your dentist.

261. There is no real evidence that teeth whitening products will harm a baby during pregnancy or nursing. You should play it safe and avoid taking any chances. There is no reason to risk your baby's health just to have a whiter smile. Go to your dentist and have a good cleaning done.

262. Rather than focusing on removing stains from your teeth with whitening pastes, creams and gels, why not avoid staining them in the first place? Coffee and tea are notorious for staining teeth and should be avoided if at all possible. If you do drink them, try rinsing your mouth out with clean water when you are done to minimize staining.

263. If you are a smoker, you are going to have a constant battle trying to keep your teeth white. If you are that worried about a white smile, you are going to need to quit or at least cut down in the amount that you are smoking. It will be a never ending battle if you continue to smoke heavily.

264. Rinse your mouth with hydrogen peroxide before you brush your teeth. This is a natural

remedy that is cheap and works well. It will help whiten your teeth and it isn't as harsh as other whitening methods. Be careful not to swallow it because it will make you sick and possibly vomit.

265.   Floss your teeth twice a day. It's best to do this to prevent plaque, which can discolor your teeth. Make sure you floss in the morning but, most importantly, before you go to sleep because this is when teeth are most susceptible to damage and plaque buildup. Flossing before you go to sleep will prevent this.

266.   Drinking through a straw is going to help you keep your teeth looking whiter longer. It will reduce the time that the drink has to settle on your teeth and cause stains. The straw will carry the drink past your teeth and closer to your throat keeping it from getting to your teeth.

267.   Make sure you regularly brush your teeth. You should make sure you brush your teeth at least two times a day, once in the morning and at night. More importantly, you should make sure you are properly brushing. This will help avoid a buildup of plaque and will help keep your teeth white.

268.   In order to get white teeth a good habit that you can do is to choose to eat food that naturally whitens teeth. Examples of these are raw fruits and vegetables that scrub your teeth while you eat them. These foods include carrots, strawberries, apples, celery, pineapples, oranges and pears.

269.   Discontinue the use of any teeth whitening products if your teeth begin to feel more sensitive. You could be damaging your teeth beyond repair. Go see your dentist for advice. Consult your dental professional to learn about what options are best for you.

270.   Invest in a set of teeth whitening trays to get the very best results while bleaching your teeth. Whitening trays are made from impressions of your teeth and are a harder plastic than the standard rubbery trays included in many whitening kits. You can get the trays from your dentist, but better yet, there are many reputable manufacturers of the trays online that are willing to send you the materials and guide you through the process of taking impressions of your own teeth at home. Simply return the impressions for a set of custom trays. Trays very effectively keep the whitening product in place, and save on the amount of product needed to do the job.

271.   Professional whitening for your teeth can provide the fastest results. A few dental visits will easily make your teeth whiter. Dentists know more about teeth whitening methods than anyone and have access to more products.

272.   When drinking beverages like coffee, soda, wines or teas, try drinking water at the same time. Those kinds of drinks are known to cause stains quickly, especially when consumed regularly. By drinking a little water with them, you will rinse off the excess residue that can cling to the teeth and stain them. If you can brush your teeth after you have finished your drink, you will also minimize any staining.

273.   When you want whiter teeth, do not be fooled by the different kinds of toothpastes available. Toothpaste that claims to whiten your teeth is frequently more expensive than normal toothpaste. When trying to remove stains from your teeth, regular toothpaste works just as well and is often cheaper than whitening toothpaste.

274.   Make appointments with your local dentist regularly to clean your teeth. There is nothing that can be as thorough as a dentist in cleaning your teeth and helping you keep a white smile. If

you have the dentist clean your teeth once or even twice a year, you will see that you have to worry less about keeping your teeth white- the only exception is unless you are a smoker.

275.   When using over-the-counter teeth whitening products it is important to read and follow the directions very carefully. Don't leave the strips or gel on longer than the instructions dictate, as this could lead to sores and problems in your mouth. Avoid drinking or eating acidic foods or beverages for a couple of hours after treatment.

276.   Do not start a home teeth whitening treatment without going to the dentist to have an exam done. You do not want to use any of these treatments if you have untreated cavities in your mouth. The same goes for gum disease. These things should be treated prior to any treatment.

277.   You can make your own whitening toothpaste with some peroxide and baking soda. Use this on your teeth for about five minutes. Be careful that you do not brush too hard, as it could cause gum irritation.

278.   Practice good oral hygiene to whiten your teeth and keep your smile bright. Brush your

teeth at least twice a day and floss regularly to remove food particles that become trapped between them. Taking good care of your teeth is one of the best ways to keep them clean, white and healthy for years to come.

279.   Store all teeth whitening products in the refrigerator to keep them as fresh as possible. Old whitening gels that have been exposed to changes in temperature can acquire an off-taste and lose their effectiveness quickly. For those with some gum sensitivities, whitening products applied right out of the refrigerator help alleviate that bit of burning sting that some products have.

280.   When you use a whitening product, it is important that you do not over do it. This can cause that natural enamel of your teeth to erode. If this happens, your teeth will become very sensitive and can become incredibly damaged. Remember that the health of your teeth should come before their appearance.

281.   Individuals who love red wine and have been drinking it for years are generally prime candidates for discolored teeth. Red wine's deep colors get absorbed into your teeth's enamel, which causes a darker hue to your teeth. The

only way to keep your teeth whiter is to stop drinking the red wine, or at least cutting back on it.

282.   The first line of defense against any type of discoloring problem is a dental regimen that includes a whitening toothpaste as well as a mouthwash to help with this. While these things alone won't be able to completely whiten your teeth they will be a very good start to give you a good base.

283.   To help prevent your teeth from getting stained, try to stay away from foods and drinks that are known to stain your teeth. Avoid foods like blueberries and soy sauce. In moderation, these foods are okay, but try not to over do it. Drinks like tea and coffee will also cause stains on your teeth.

284.   A great way to naturally whiten your teeth without resorting to harsh chemicals is to use a baking soda and salt mixture. This is a method that has been used by many people for a long time, that is both safe and cost effective. There are plenty of toothpaste products that use baking soda in them.

285.   Use whitening toothpaste. Any kind of toothpaste is a whitener but a toothpaste with a whitening agent in it will speed up the process. Regular flossing of your teeth will also prevent stains from plaque before they occur. Both will help keep your teeth whiter for a longer time period.

286.   A great tip that can help you whiten your teeth is to brush your teeth right after you have your cup of coffee. It's no secret that coffee is known to stain teeth. A trick that can prevent stains from occurring is to simply brush your teeth after drinking coffee. Wy not carry a mini toothcare set with you?

287.   Stop any tooth whitening technique immediately if you notice your teeth becoming more sensitive or if they begin to develop spots or stains. Most teeth whitening remedies do not harm the teeth, but there is always a possibility the enamel may become damaged. Increasing sensitivity or discoloration is an early indicator of damage and should warn you to stop any whitening technique.

288.   If you're a pregnant or lactating mother, you should not undergo any teeth whitening procedure. It can have many negative effects on

the baby. Before having your teeth whitened, you should consult with your dentist and let them know up front if you're pregnant or lactating. They'll be able to say for sure whether it's a danger to the baby or not.

289.   Using baking soda is one of the oldest and best ways to whiten your teeth. Take your baking soda in a small container and mix it with water to make a paste type solution. Use it to brush your teeth and then follow up and rinse with peroxide and brush with toothpaste!

290.   Use natural tooth whiteners, such as baking soda, orange peels, or lemon peels. Mixing any of these with a little salt can make an excellent cheap tooth whitening product. Be sure to wash your mouth out thoroughly after using any of these methods, as the harsh acids can damage your teeth.

291.   Be sure that the teeth whitening trays fit your mouth correctly. If they do not fit well there is a good chance that they are going to cause you problems with your gums. If you notice that your gums are more sensitive or in any pain, stop using the product and see your dentist.

292.   Increase the amount of foods in your diet that clean your teeth. These include high-fiber fruits and vegetables such as carrots, apples, celery, and cauliflower. These work to whiten your teeth by scrubbing off plaque as you eat. They also cause your mouth to produce more saliva, which results in healthier enamel and whiter teeth.

293.   Rinse your mouth with hydrogen peroxide before you brush your teeth. This is a natural remedy that is cheap and works well. It will help whiten your teeth and it isn't as harsh as other whitening methods. Be careful not to swallow it because it will make you sick and possibly vomit.

294.   Once you go through the teeth whitening treatment, you are going to want to avoid drinking things or eating foods that are known to stain teeth. Newly whitened teeth are prone to absorbing the staining agents that are in these things and you may find yourself worse off than before you treated your teeth.

295.   Read as many reviews about whitening products as you can before buying one. If you take the time to research the products before you spend your money on them, you are sure to find

a quality product a lot quicker and without spending as much money.

296.   For inexpensive teeth whitening at home, brush your teeth thoroughly and then swish a mouthful of hydrogen peroxide inside your mouth for as long as possible before spitting it out into the sink. Hydrogen peroxide is an active ingredient in most commercial teeth whitening products and provides an oxygenating action that helps lift stains from teeth.

297.   If you're considering having your teeth whitened, talk to your dentist first. While some stains and discoloration are easily treated by bleaching, others won't respond as well. Bleaching also won't work if you have caps, crowns, or similar types of dental work. Discussing teeth whitening with your dentist will prepare you for potential problems and help you figure out the best way to treat your teeth.

298.   When you decide to do any kind of dental regimen that includes whitening your teeth you should be sure to have the advice of a dental professional. If you try to do things completely on your own you may make amateur mistakes that will set back your progress by several months.

299.   Many people give up coffee and move to tea in an attempt to have whiter teeth. While this has not been proven to actually whiten teeth it will certainly help to prevent further discoloring. This is because coffee is one of the worst things you can do to the color of your teeth.

300.   Whiter teeth can happen by simply eliminating odors in your mouth. You can lick your clean palm to test your breath. If it smells, use mouthwash or a breath mint. Always be certain that your mouthwash is free of alcohol, as it can have a drying effect.

301.   A great at-home product that you can use to get whiter teeth is a strawberry. The natural ingredients in strawberries have been proven to whiten teeth. You can cut the strawberry in half and use the part without the stem to rub on your teeth. Rinse it off after 5 minutes.

302.   Enamel protects your teeth from harmful infections and cavities. There are some products for sale that are not good for your teeth, so try not to purchase anything that contains high acidity or toxic chemicals. Read product reviews online before purchasing for further information.

303.   There are a few herbs that have teeth-whitening properties. These include: holy basil, margosa, banyon roots and babul. You can rub these herbs directly on your front teeth to whiten them, or you can mix them with a paste of baking soda and water or mashed-up strawberries and then apply to your teeth.

304.   In order to get your teeth as white as possible, you may want to talk to your dentist about Luma-light or Zoom treatments. These treatments have a high concentration of peroxide with light wavelengths, and is so effective, that your teeth could end up 10 shades lighter. It is also a safe procedure.

305.   Going to a dentist and paying to have your teeth bleached is very effective. Bleaching solution is applied to the teeth and it stays there for about an hour. Do not worry about taste or burns because they take precautions to prevent this from happening to you. Results can usually be seen after just one session.

306.   Before the invention of fancy teeth whitening mouthwashes and toothpastes, baking soda served as a great alternative. You can still use baking soda to effectively whiten your teeth. Pour some baking soda on your toothbrush and

start brushing your teeth. Make sure that you do not swallow the baking soda and rinse out thoroughly when finished. You can easily see the whitening effects within the first few weeks.

307.   If you drink dark wine, coffee, soda or tea, try alternating your consumption with sips of water. These can stain quickly, especially if consumed regularly. Rinsing or sipping water following imbibing them can remove residual residue that creates stains. Also, be sure to brush after.

308.   Heavy smoking can in fact damage and stain your teeth. It helps to cut down on the amount of cigarettes you smoke each day or eliminate them out of your life completely. People who smoke have a harder time keeping their teeth clean than those who don't.

309.   Rinse your mouth out after drinking coffee or tea. They are both well known for staining teeth. For better results, try to eliminate it from your diet altogether. The same goes for soda and wine; they can stain your teeth just as much, if not more than coffee and tea.

310.   Use baking soda to brush your teeth instead of regular toothpaste. This is a popular home

remedy. Baking soda acts as a mild detergent for the teeth. When using baking soda to brush your teeth, be gentle in order to avoid gum irritation.

311.   When using over-the-counter teeth whitening products it is important to read and follow the directions very carefully. Don't leave the strips or gel on longer than the instructions dictate, as this could lead to sores and problems in your mouth. Avoid drinking or eating acidic foods or beverages for a couple of hours after treatment.

312.   Mix baking soda and salt together for an at-home whitening method. This is a well known treatment for making teeth whiter. You can make a paste out of it by mixing them together with a little bit of water. Make sure you rinse your mouth out well afterwards.

313.   Use whitening strips. Depending on how badly your teeth are stained, they usually don't immediately work. Over time, you will notice your teeth getting whiter. You should use these strips regularly, but not too much. These strips are easy and convenient to use and keep you from visiting the dentist.

314.   When using over the counter teeth whitening products, make sure that you follow the instructions exactly. Some people may try to leave strips or gels on their teeth longer than directed in an effort to enhance or quicken results. This can cause irritation to your gums and result in inflammation. Stick to the directions and exercise patience.

315.   One of the primary causes of having discolored teeth and smile in general is bad habits with beverages. Coffee is one of the leading causes of having teeth that are discolored. If you are determined to continue drinking coffee then you will want to brush your teeth immediately after each cup.

316.   It can sometimes be good to use a toothpaste designed for whitening. While whitening toothpastes lack the power of other whitening methods, they can still be very effective in the prevention and treatment of stains. Whitening toothpastes scrub at stains and discoloration with silica abrasives, which are strong enough to be effective, but not so strong that you wear down your enamel.

317.   You can change the look of your smile by simply changing your lipstick color. You should

wear lipstick that has a blue base or just simply use a gloss. Hues like berry shades and blue-tinted reds are very effective at making your teeth seem whiter. You should not wear lipstick that is matte colored as it will make your smile appear more tarnished and yellow.

318.   If you want your teeth to be whiter, you need to get your teeth cleaned regularly. Setting and keeping a regular cleaning schedule is a powerful tool in your teeth-whitening toolbox. Dental cleanings should be on your schedule semiannually.

319.   Brush and floss at least a twice a day. This will help to prevent a buildup of plaque, which can discolor your teeth. It is also a good idea to carry floss with you, that way you can floss anytime after you eat. Paying special attention to your teeth will help to prevent staining.

320.   Surprisingly, you will have less discoloration of your teeth if you stop using mouthwash. Since mouthwash contains chemicals including alcohol, it can stain your teeth with brown and yellow stains, because it strips the enamel. Talk to your dentist about whether your teeth can withstand the damage that mouthwash causes.

321.	Don't use mouthwashes. If your teeth are not getting whiter despite your efforts, consider doing way with your mouthwash altogether. Mouthwashes are made with a host of different chemical ingredients. Some of the ingredients can stain your teeth.

322.	Add parsley and cilantro to your daily meals for a natural herbal teeth whitener. These foods offer a natural way to fight germs and bacteria that can discolor teeth. However, remember to also use toothpaste on a regular basis.